THE NEW LIFE LIBRARY
# REFLEXOLOGY

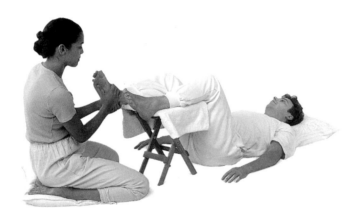

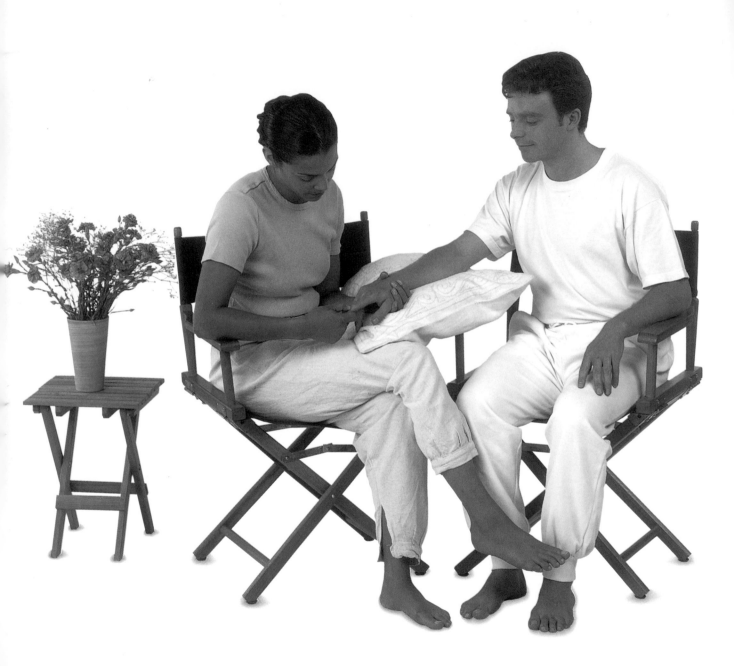

THE NEW LIFE LIBRARY

# REFLEXOLOGY

## SIMPLE TECHNIQUES TO RELIEVE STRESS
## AND ENHANCE YOUR MIND

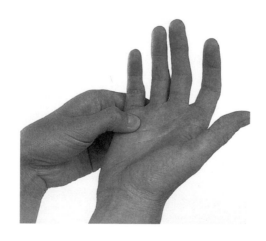

## ROSALIND OXENFORD

LORENZ BOOKS
LONDON • NEW YORK • SYDNEY • BATH

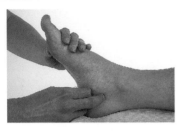

This edition published in the UK in 1997
by Lorenz Books.

This edition published in the USA in 1997 by
Lorenz Books, 27 West 20th Street
New York, NY 10011.

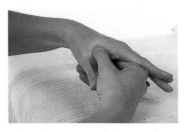

Lorenz Books are available for bulk purchase for sales promotion and for premium use. For details write or call the manager of special sales, Lorenz Books, 27 West 20th Street, New York, NY 10011; (212) 807 6739.

ISBN 1 85967 342 2

*Publisher: Joanna Lorenz*
*Editorial Manager: Helen Sudell*
*Designer: Bobbie Colgate Stone*
*Photographer: Don Last*
*Illustrator: Michael Shoebridge*
*Models: Elizabeth Alvey, Georgia Daniels, Jonathan May, Diana Wilson*

3 5 7 9 10 8 6 4 2

Printed and bound in China

Publisher's note: The reader should not regard the recommendations, ideas and techniques expressed and described in this book as substitutes for the advice of a qualified medical practitioner or other qualified professional. Any use to which the recommendations, ideas and techniques are put is at the reader's sole discretion and risk.

# CONTENTS

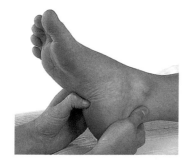

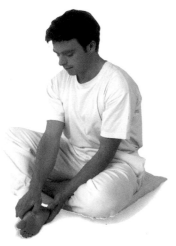

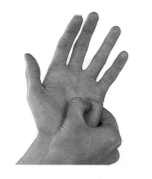

# INTRODUCTION

USING OUR HANDS to release tension in our bodies is something we do instinctively. When you bang your shin it is an automatic response to hold your hurt leg or rub it better. You are thus releasing the disturbed energy from the traumatized part of your body through contact with the undisturbed energy of your hands. In effect you are re-balancing the traumatized part to restore it to its natural state of well-being, with harmony between the flow of energy, circulation and muscle tension.

Our hands have been a means of caring, comfort and giving since we first ceased to need them to walk on and started to use them for focused, specialized activities. They are the tools of many natural therapies. In reflexology

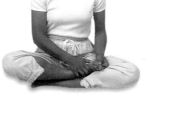

Above: Reflexology is useful as a means of self-help.

you can use them, specifically your fingers, to apply pressure-point therapy to certain points: usually on the feet, often on the hands. There are reflex points elsewhere, notably on the head, but these are used less frequently.

The word "reflex" means to reflect. Pressure points on your feet and hands reflect all the parts of your body, both external and internal: organs and glands as well as limbs, torso and head. Each point reflects the activity of another part of the body. In conventional medicine a reflex is a spontaneous action in response to a stimulus received by a nerve, the message being relayed to the spinal column and back to the body part without reference to the brain, as, for instance, when you drop something that is too hot to touch. This is a direct communication through the nervous system. In reflexology, as in acupuncture, places or points relate to or reflect organs of the body, but not in such an apparently direct way as this.

In physics, the science of the properties of matter and energy and the basis of all natural science, the behaviour and movement of energy is clearly understood. This applies equally to our bodies, as we are part of the natural world and subject to its laws. In natural medicine the energy within us is known as the life force or vital energy. In China it is called Chi, in India Prana, in Japan Ki.

# THE HISTORY OF REFLEXOLOGY

Treatment of the feet and hands and of pressure points has been practised for thousands of years, the earliest known evidence being a relief in a mastaba (funerary monument) at Saqqara in Egypt dated around 2,500-2,300 BC (see bottom right). The tomb was that of two priests of the royal palace, during the 5th Dynasty of the Pharaohs.

The feet were worked in ancient China in conjunction with acupuncture, the feet being treated first to stimulate the whole body and find areas of disturbance, and acupuncture needles then being applied as fine tuning. Foot treatment was also practised in India and Indonesia and among native Americans, who hold a central belief that our feet are our connection with the earth and the earth's energies.

In Europe pressure-point therapy was used from the Middle Ages onwards, but it was not until this century that enquiring Westerners brought together the wisdom and practices of ancient cultures with a modern understanding of the subject. Notable among these are Dr William Fitzgerald, who noticed that pressure on points of the body affected other parts lying along the same line or zone within the body, and Eunice Ingham, who first mapped out the specific reflex points on the feet. Robert St John was the first to explore the psychological as well as the physiological effects of treatment, and Inge Dougans worked to show the links in understanding between what is now termed reflexology and meridian theory, which we know most about through acupuncture and the Law of the Five Elements (the principles and understanding of Traditional Chinese Acupuncture).

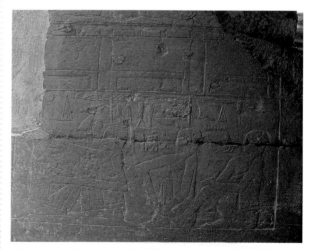

Above: An Egyptian relief from the tomb of two priests of the royal palace during the 5th Dynasty, dated around 2,500-2,300 BC. It shows two men treating two other men, one working on the hands and the other on the feet.

# HOW REFLEXOLOGY WORKS

Reflexology acts on parts of the body by stimulating the corresponding reflexes with compression techniques applied with the fingers. Where there is inhibited functioning, or disease, we find congestion in the form of deposits that have not been cleared away by the venous circulation and the lymph.

Places on the feet where there are congestion deposits will feel tender, sensitive or positively painful; or they may feel hard, tight or lumpy, or like little grains. If these can be worked with massage and compression techniques so that they begin to disperse, the corresponding body part will be stimulated and enabled to heal itself.

## HOW THE BODY FITS ON TO THE FEET

Both feet together hold the reflexes to the whole body. The part that corresponds to the spine therefore runs down the medial line along the instep (the inner edge) of each foot. It will be useful to refer to the charts at the back of the book when reading this section, as they show a picture of the inside body parts in each area of the feet.

Right: Working on the spinal reflex that runs along the instep of each foot.

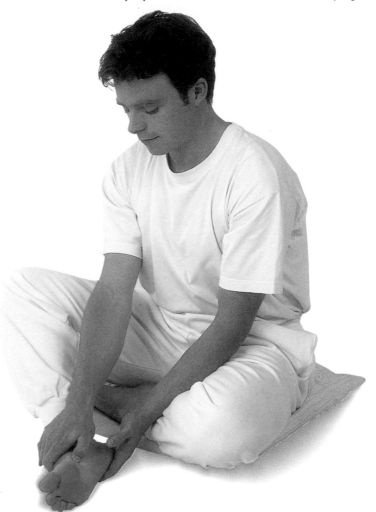

## HEAD AND NECK

Your head is represented on the toes; the right side of your head lies on the right big toe and the left side on the left big toe. In addition to the whole head being fully represented on the two big toes, the eight little toes hold the reflexes to specific parts of your head, for fine tuning.

Your neck reflex is found in the "necks" of all the toes: if you find tension in one area of your neck, you will find tension or discomfort, or be able to feel congestion, in the corresponding areas of your toes. The correspondence between the head and toes may be difficult to understand at first because you have only one head and ten toes (or only two sides to your head and five toes on either side).

## TORSO AND SPINE

It is much easier to comprehend how the torso fits on to the body of the feet once you have grasped the concept of your two feet together representing your whole body. Remember that the spinal line runs down the insteps of your feet, where they meet if you put them together.

## ZONES ON THE FEET

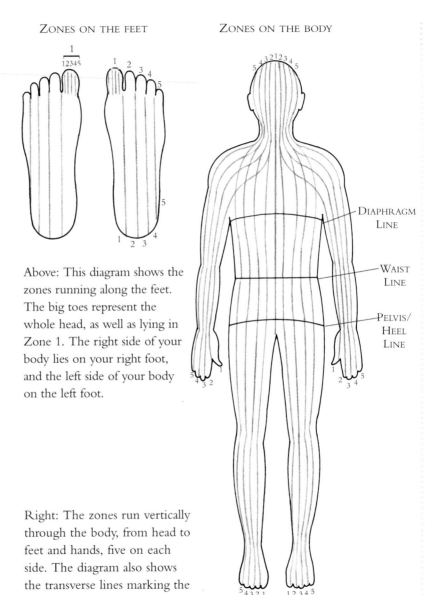

Above: This diagram shows the zones running along the feet. The big toes represent the whole head, as well as lying in Zone 1. The right side of your body lies on your right foot, and the left side of your body on the left foot.

## ZONES ON THE BODY

DIAPHRAGM LINE

WAIST LINE

PELVIS/ HEEL LINE

Right: The zones run vertically through the body, from head to feet and hands, five on each side. The diagram also shows the transverse lines marking the areas of the body.

9

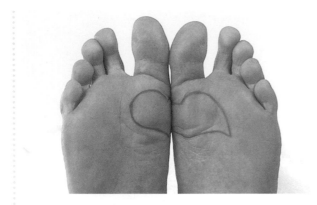

### CHEST
The ball of each foot represents one side of your chest. So in the balls of your feet, and on the same area on the top of your feet, lie the reflexes to your lungs, air passages, heart, thymus gland, breast, shoulders and everything contained in your chest. The whole area is bounded by your diaphragm, the important reflex that lies across the base of the ball of each foot.

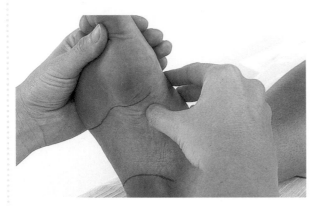

### ABDOMEN
In your instep, where your feet are not weight-bearing and so not padded like the ball, are contained all the reflexes to your abdominal organs - those concerned with digestion and the maintenance of life. This area is bounded by the diaphragm line above and by the heel line below.

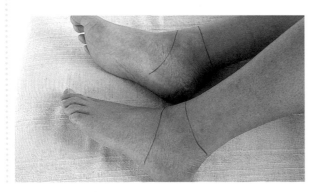

### PELVIS
The whole of your heel all around your foot contains the reflexes to your pelvic area: they lie on the sole and the sides of your heel and across the top of your ankle.

10

LIMBS

The limbs are represented on the outer edge of your foot but also, and most particularly, on the corresponding upper or lower limb. There is no part of the foot that resembles the limbs, whereas you can see fairly easily how the head corresponds to the toes and the torso to the body of the foot. Arms and legs, however, follow the same basic structure and each limb holds the reflexes to the other limb on the same side. These are called cross reflexes.

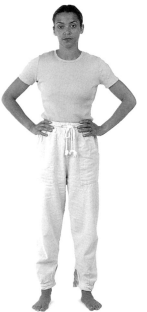

Shoulders reflect hips, and hips reflect shoulders, so you can work your shoulder for hip problems and vice versa.

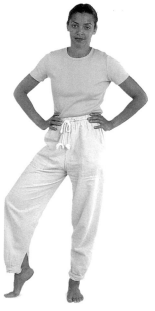

In the same way, elbows and knees relate to each other.

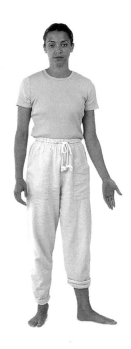

Work the wrist for ankle problems, and vice versa.

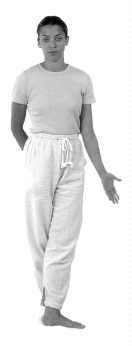

Hand and foot are cross reflexes for each other.

# THE BENEFITS AND EFFECTS OF REFLEXOLOGY

Reflexology works to relax muscle tension. During a treatment all parts of the feet are stimulated to relax muscles and increase the circulation to all parts of the body. The immediate effect of this is to achieve a deep state of relaxation.

Working along holistic principles, reflexology takes into account body, mind and spirit as these are all interrelated. Whatever happens to you will affect all levels of your being, whether you notice or not. If you feel under pressure or stressed, the effect on your body will be detrimental as your muscles remain tense and taut, constricting the circulation and nerves, and compromising their functioning. Similarly, if you have a physical mishap your feelings will be affected by the pain you experience, the way the accident happened, and the effect it has on you afterwards.

Although you are working mostly on the feet in reflexology, you are affecting the whole of the

Above: Through working the hands (or feet) you are working the whole body.

body, both inside and out, through the treatment. This is achieved by working the reflexes to the internal organs and glands as well as to the surface of the body. It appears that you can have a more far-reaching effect by working the reflexes than by working directly on the corresponding body part.

Pain in the back, for instance, may be due to a structural problem in which the bones are actually out of place and should be checked by a cranial osteopath, osteopath or chiropractor. If the pain results from muscular problems, or if manipulation has already been done but muscular strain remains, the next step is to identify the muscles involved and work to relieve the situation with massage and reflexology.

Massage has an immediate and profoundly relieving effect, but the pain and discomfort is likely to recur when the effects of the massage have worn off. Longer term benefits result from working the reflexes to the relevant area of the back than from working directly on those muscles concerned. This is because through the reflexes you are stimulating the body from within, rather than exercising and

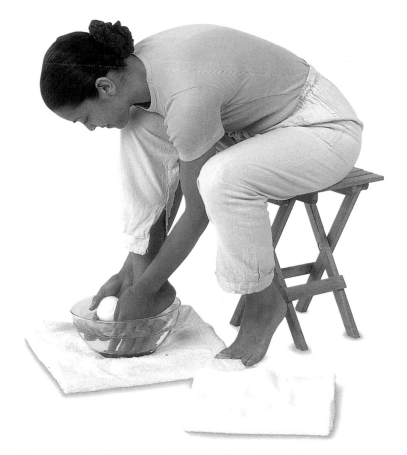

Above: It is advisable to wash your feet thoroughly before any treatment to cleanse and refresh the skin.

soothing the muscles from without. Stimulating the reflex to a troubled area will promote healing. Reflexology uses both massage and specific stimulation of the reflexes to gain lasting relief.

WHAT A TREATMENT INVOLVES
Reflexology is not foot massage, but this is incorporated. Sweeping whole hand movements on the whole foot will relax the entire person and prepare the feet for

reflex work. During the working of the reflexes, massage soothes and relaxes the area where congestion or discomfort is found. It links the treatment together into a continuous whole and relaxes and stimulates the whole body while individual parts are being treated specifically. Equally beneficial is the use of whole hand massage movements to complete a reflexology treatment and to give a feeling of well-being to the entire person before ending the treatment.

A reflexology session can be both relaxing and stimulating for the patient. As muscle tensions are relaxed, and the nerve supply freed from constriction, the body slips into a deep state of relaxation. At the same time, the circulation is being stimulated to bring nutrients to all parts of the body and to remove waste products and toxins that interfere with the healthy functioning of the parts and the whole. Energy is able to flow more freely and fully around the body, the functioning of the various systems is thus optimized and feelings of well-being result.

### THE EFFECTS: WHAT YOU MAY FEEL LIKE AFTER REFLEXOLOGY TREATMENT

Some people find that they feel relaxed and sleepy for some time after a reflexology session; they may feel very tired and need to rest for a while. Many others feel deeply relaxed at the end of a session but find that when they leave, or soon afterwards, they feel energized and motivated.

### TOXINS AND THE HEALING REACTION

Waste products are formed in the body as a result of muscular activity; others are the result of your intake of processed food, additives, drugs or any other substances that your body recognizes as alien or unwanted. Included in this group of waste products that the body finds toxic are the by-products of stress as well as those of routine muscular processes.

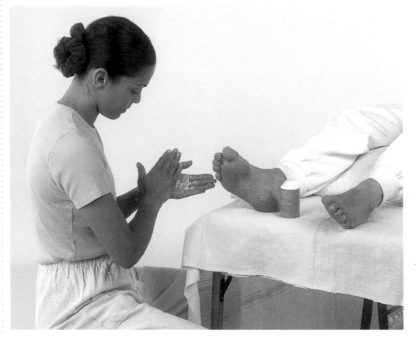

Above: A little powder lightly dusted on to your hands will prevent them from sticking while working on the feet.

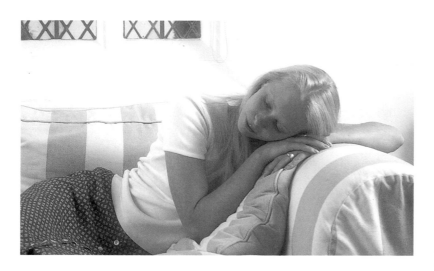

Left: You may feel deeply relaxed after a reflexology treatment.

These healing reactions will pass in hours, or at most in a couple of days, as the body finds a new equilibrium. If, following reflexology, discomfort or illness occurs that does not represent a loosening of the body and evidence of improved functioning, then it is likely to have nothing to do with the treatment and a doctor should be consulted.

Where there are many waste products to be cleared, you may experience a healing reaction (sometimes referred to as a healing crisis) to treatment, which will rid the body or mind of unwanted substances. It may take the form of a runny nose, increased perspiration or urination, or increased bowel movements. You may feel emotional or dream more if the unwanted "substances" are feelings, or even suffer from a headache when feelings can find no other mode of expression. Whatever the reaction, it will be a "throwing off" and will represent a loosening of body tensions and evidence of improved functioning.

## CAUTION

If you choose to use this book to try reflexology yourself, it is imperative that you do so only when the person receiving it is in good health. If you know someone who is ill and who would like to receive reflexology, they should be treated by a recognized and accredited practitioner. A professional reflexologist will never treat someone without first checking on their medical condition and background, and when there is any illness or disorder will advise that the client consult their doctor before proceeding.
If you wish to give reflexology to someone who does not have any medical condition but who does not seem to be well, or who has one of the everyday "first-aid" discomforts described in the sequences in this book, it is again imperative that if they seem at all worryingly unwell they should receive professional help before you do anything at all. If you are subsequently able to give some reflexology you must still proceed with great caution to safeguard both of you from mishap.

# PREPARATION

Make sure the room you are going to use is warm and that you may be quiet in there without interruptions from the telephone, people coming in and going out, or restless pets.

Find a comfortable position for the person whose feet you are going to be treating. They may be propped up along a sofa, with cushions to support their back, head and neck in one corner, and their feet at the opposite front edge of the sofa so that you can reach them. If they are sitting in an armchair, find an upright chair or stool of a suitable height to support their legs, with a cushion underneath them. Alternatively, you can position your partner on the floor (see right). Make sure that their back, neck and head are fully supported so as not to place the spine under any strain, and that the knees are bent so that the circulation can flow freely: do not work with the knees straight.

If your partner has sore feet and you are going to work on their hands, it is probably easier to learn the reflexes if you sit side by side rather than opposite each other. In this way the hands will be the same way up as when you are

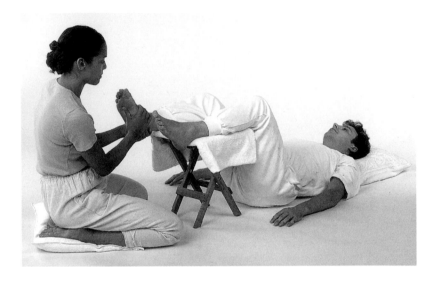

Above: The feet must be where you can comfortably reach them.

Right: Support your arms comfortably while you do reflexology on your hands. Being comfortable will help you to relax.

working on your own hands.

To work on your own feet or hands, find a position that is comfortable for you.

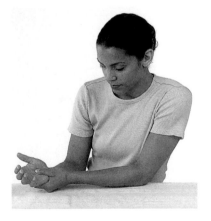

## EQUIPMENT

Whichever position you use, you will need to have plenty of pillows to support the back, neck and head. A pillow should be placed under your partner's knees so that they are bent.

Have a blanket or cover ready in case your partner needs extra warmth - their body temperature may drop as they relax.

You will need some towels: one to place under the feet and one or two more for the foot you are not working on to cover it and keep it warm.

Have some powder or arrowroot in case you find that your hands stick to the skin of the feet as you work, if much heat or moisture is released.

Arrange a pile of cushions, a big cushion or a low stool to sit on as you work. You need to be able to reach and see the feet comfortably without bending over from too high above them. It is very important that you are comfortable: becoming strained or tired will not be good for you, and you may not pay attention properly as you work and could risk doing some damage to your partner.

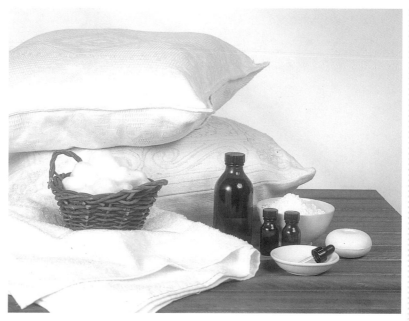

Have pillows, towels, cotton wool, powder, soap and oils handy.

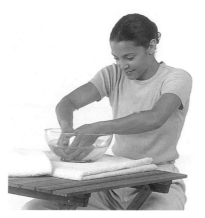

Before you begin, wash the feet or hands in soap and water.

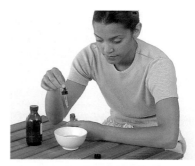

Alternatively, if you have and use essential oils, use a small bowl of water and add a couple of drops of lavender and one of tea tree oil to cleanse them.

# WARM-UP FOOT MASSAGE

It is of great benefit to the patient if the feet are massaged at the beginning of a reflexology treatment to introduce your patient to your touch. You should also massage in between specific reflex work, and also to complete the treatment at the end.

### TO BEGIN

Massage prepares the feet for reflex work: it warms and relaxes the tissues, accustoms the receiver to your touch and soothes and relaxes the whole body. Massage will loosen tensions in the muscles and stimulate the blood supply to and around the feet so that when the reflex points are worked the tissues will not be strained and they can respond fully.

### DURING TREATMENT

Use plenty of massage to link the movement from one reflex area to the next, to soothe and relax the foot in between working the reflex points, which may produce sensations of tenderness, and use it where any tenderness or discomfort is found.

### TO COMPLETE

When you have covered all the reflex points, do not just stop, as this could leave your partner feeling fragmented. It is much more pleasant to end with some whole hand massage on both feet to round the treatment off and instil a sense of well-being and relaxation. At this point you may use 2-3 drops of essential oil mixed in almond oil, which will feel flowing and nurturing. Do not use oils in massage until you have completed the reflex work, as your hands will slide around and not be accurate.

### THE MASSAGE MOVEMENTS

There is no set sequence for these movements. When you have learnt them, fit them together in a way that feels good to you and adapt them for the individual you are working with as you feel is appropriate. The first few are good as an introduction, and you should always rotate the ankles as this frees up the blood and nerve supply through the ankle to the foot.

### EFFLEURAGE OR STROKING

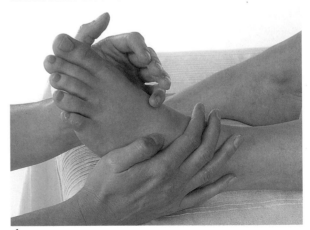

**1** These movements are just as they sound – sweeping and soothing – and are good to do all over the foot. Add some effleurage wherever it feels appropriate throughout the treatment.

SPREADING MOVEMENTS

Use these to relax the muscles and stimulate the circulation.

ANKLE ROTATION

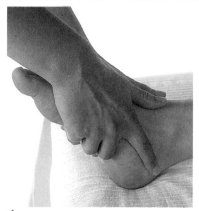

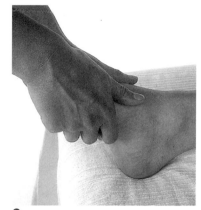

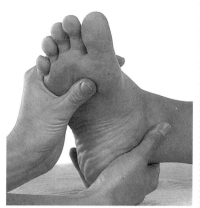

**1** For the top of the foot, draw your thumbs off sideways, keeping your fingers still.

**2** Repeat the first movement, working your way down the foot with each repetition.

**1** Rotate the foot clockwise several times, feeling as you go so that you do not force stiff ankles but you do exercise the joint.

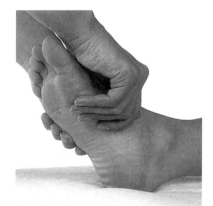

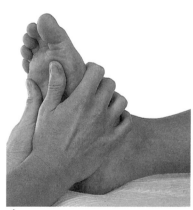

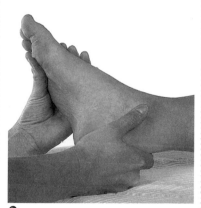

**3** To cover the sole of the foot, start in the same position as before, but this time draw your fingers off sideways, keeping your thumbs still.

**4** Finally, massage into the ball of the foot with your thumbs.

**2** Repeat the ankle rotation in an anti-clockwise direction.

KNEADING

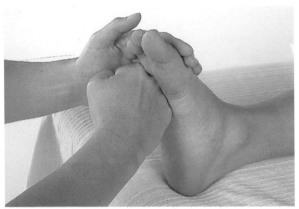

**1** Using a similar movement to kneading bread dough, work into the sole of the foot using the lower section of your fingers, not your knuckles. Use your other hand to support the front of the foot, as shown.

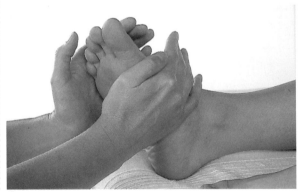

**2** With your hands in the same starting position, this time move them alternately up and down from the top to the sole of the foot so that the foot tips from side to side. Take care not to twist the ankle.

VIGOROUS, FAST MOVEMENTS

These are used to stimulate sluggish tissues or help to bring a sleepy person "back to earth" at the end of a treatment. In all these movements your two hands move in opposite directions to one another.

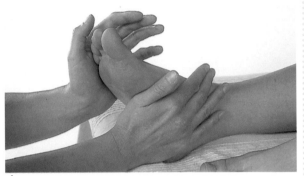

**1** Massage the sides of the foot, running your hands up and down the length of the foot.

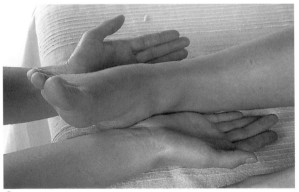

**3** With your hands palms up on either side of the foot, move them quickly to and fro, to exercise and loosen the ankle. When this movement is done correctly, the foot will waggle around.

TOE ROTATION

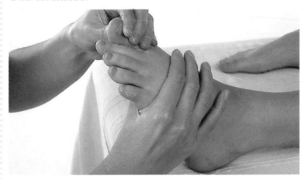

Beginning with the big toe, hold the toe securely (but not too tightly) and gently rotate. Repeat the movement with each toe.

TO RELAX THE DIAPHRAGM

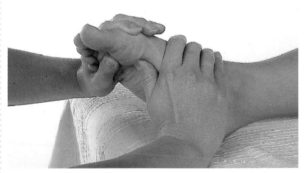

This movement is rather like drawing beer from a traditional hand pump. Hold the foot with your outside hand (the one nearest the little toe), bring the foot down on to the thumb of your other hand and lift it off again. Next, move your thumb one step to the side and repeat the movement. Repeat until you have worked along the boundary line of the ball of the foot where it meets the instep (the diaphragm line).

SPINAL TWIST

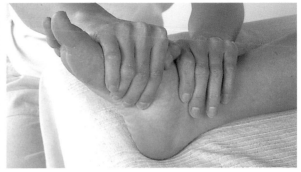

The hand on the ankle remains still while the other, lower hand moves to and fro across the top of the foot, round the instep and back again.

TO ESTABLISH GOOD BREATHING AND RELAX THE SOLAR PLEXUS REFLEX

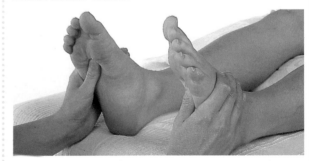

Take both feet together and position your thumbs in the centre of the diaphragm line where there is a natural dent, or place that "gives" when you press gently. Ask your partner to breathe in and then to release the breath. As they breathe in, press gently in with your thumbs and as they breathe out, release your thumbs. Repeat this several times following your partner's lead so that the rhythm is comfortable for them.

# REFLEXOLOGY TECHNIQUES

## GIVING REFLEXOLOGY

Reflexology works on the whole of the body, stimulating the reflexes to the internal organs, glands and body parts, as well as massaging the outside of the body. Through working on the feet as a whole, healing is stimulated throughout the body rather than just in one part that may well be influenced, or have

influence on, other parts or systems. This is what makes the holistic approach of natural medicine so effective.

When you have a problem, natural therapies do not address you as a machine - repairing or replacing the part that does not work, regardless of its purpose in the functioning of the whole - but treat you in your

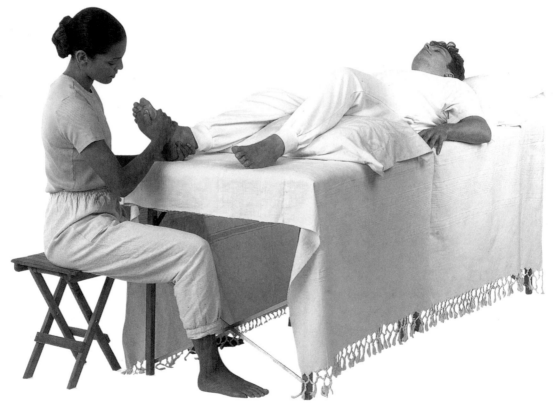

Make sure your partner is comfortable, with pillows under their head, neck and knees acting as support.

entirety to deal with the cause of the problem, rather than merely alleviating the symptoms locally. If you have a raging toothache you may be able to relieve it by taking painkillers, but you will not cause the abscess to go away unless you deal with the poison that gave rise to it in the first place.

If you develop a headache you may or may not know its cause. Where in your body is the trouble seated? Does it come from tension in your neck or lower down your spine, from digestive disturbance, or even from held-in tension in your legs? Many headaches have such roots even though we do not notice the beginning of the trouble until the pounding in our head attracts our attention. Recurrent headaches happen because their causes have not been recognized and dealt with. The headache does not really go away, even if temporarily relieved by taking painkillers.

If you were to gently massage the reflexes to the head you might be able to give temporary relief from the pain, but you will probably not get rid of the headache. Pressing a reflex point for pain relief is helpful, but short-lived. Stimulating a related reflex, usually more than one, which shows congestion or imbalance, on the other hand, is highly effective in the long term. You will only be able to find these if you work the whole of the feet, rather than spot-working for a specific symptom.

In fact, it is quite possible to make a headache worse by stimulating the reflexes to the head, as pressure is already intense there and needs to be relieved lower down, especially on the spinal column, so that it can drain away.

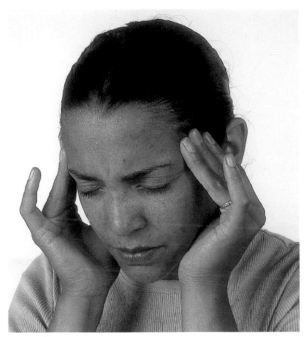

As with a headache, the actual cause of a particular problem may not lie where the pain is located.

## CAUTION

Picking out certain reflexes in isolation is only really effective in the context of working the whole. If you learn and use the routine that follows you will be able to use the sequences in the next section to great effect as part of a reflexology treatment. If you try to bring about a change using only the sequences, you are likely, at best, to be disappointed in the results and, at worst, to aggravate the problem.

## FIVE BASIC HAND TECHNIQUES
### THUMBWALKING

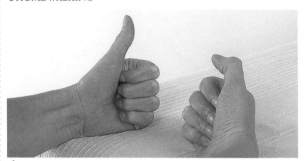

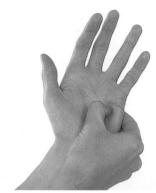

**1** Hold your two thumbs straight up in front of you and bend one at a time at the first joint. Thumbwalking is this movement repeatedly performed while the thumb rests on the skin and travels along its surface.

**2** The therapeutic movement is on the downward press with your thumb bent. As you press and move forward along the surface, put emphasis on pressing down on the skin. Use one hand only: the other holds and supports the foot or hand you are working on.

### ROTATING

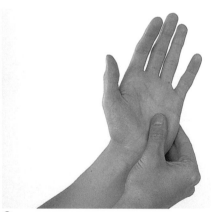

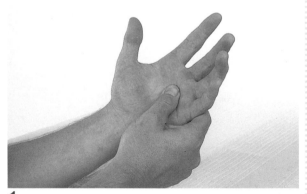

**3** Slide or skate forward as you straighten your thumb. You will still put some pressure on the surface and maintain contact but you are primarily involved in moving forward. The thumbwalking technique is sometimes called caterpillar walking.

**1** Place your thumb (or finger) on a part of your hand or foot and gently rotate it on the spot. Try exerting a little more pressure. Use this technique when you want to work a specific small point.

FINGERWALKING
This technique is the same as thumbwalking, but using one or more fingers.

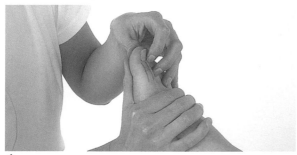

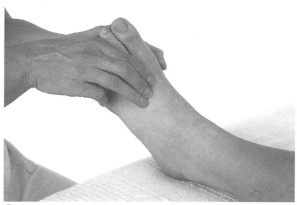

**1** Fingerwalking with the index finger.

**2** Fingerwalking with the three middle fingers together.

PINPOINTING

HOLDING AND SUPPORT

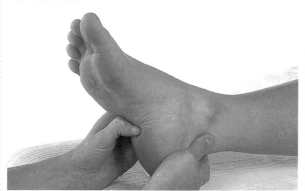

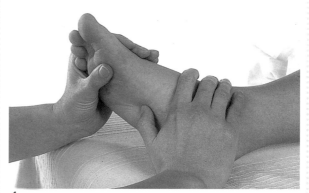

**1** Pinpointing is used only for deep or less accessible reflexes that you cannot usually reach by rotating. You use your thumb and fingers in conjunction. With your hand in mid-air, move thumb and fingers together and then apart like a pincer. Now place your hand on the foot or hand and, with the inner corner of your thumb, press deeply down into the tissues. Do this on a well-padded part, or it might hurt the receiver.

**1** Always use one hand to hold the foot or hand you are working on securely, both to give a feeling of security to your partner and to help yourself to do the techniques properly and sensitively. Position your holding hand near the working hand, not at the other end of the foot, as this can feel insecure.

# THE FULL REFLEXOLOGY ROUTINE

The following pages are a step-by-step illustration of the full reflexology routine, which should be performed on your partner before moving to treat specific problem areas. It is good to treat the areas of the body in the same order as outlined here. For easy reference to the areas described, refer to diagram of the routine below. Occasionally, lines have been drawn on the hands and feet in the photographs to highlight key reflex points.

### SUGGESTED ORDER FOR REFLEXOLOGY ROUTINE

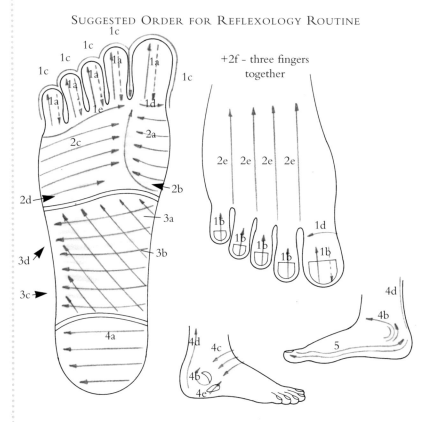

## MASSAGE

Remember to begin with some massage and to incorporate massage movements into the whole routine, between every area and when you find a tender place. Give a good thorough massage at the end to complete.

## LEFT AND RIGHT

The routine is described for one foot. Begin with the right foot and, when you have completed it, move to the left foot and duplicate what you have done (reversing hands and movements as appropriate to the shape of the left foot). At the end of the routine you will have followed the diagram on both feet. In the diagram (left) each number (ie. area of the body) has subsections marked by letters and the arrows indicate the direction of movement.

This diagram illustrates the order of reflex areas to follow to work the full reflexology routine. Refer to the diagram as often as necessary.

THE SPINE
The spine runs along the instep.
Start or finish with this routine.

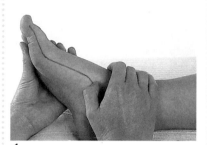

**1** Thumbwalk up the spinal line.

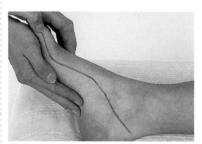

**2** Thumbwalk down the spinal line.

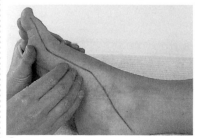

**3** Use the three middle fingers to fingerwalk across the spine/instep in stages, from big toe to heel.

THE TOES
The toes refer to the head and neck.

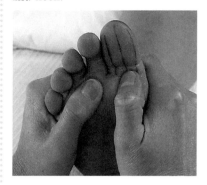

**1** Work up the back of the big toe, thumbwalking it in three lines, to cover the whole area.

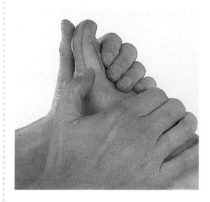

**3** Next, work up the side of the big toe with your thumb.

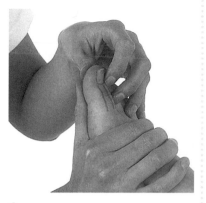

**2** Using your index finger, finger-walk down the front of the big toe, again in three lines.

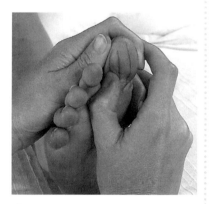

**4** For the other side of the toe, approach it from the back and tuck your thumb in between this toe and the second one before you start to thumbwalk the line up the side of the neck.  ▶

27

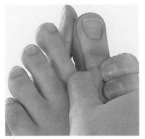

**5** Change hands and, using your other thumb, approach from the front and tuck it in between the big toe and second toe again. Work up this side to the top.

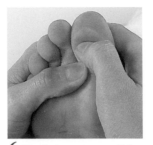

**6** Find the centre of the whorls of the big toe print and position your hand for pinpointing the pituitary reflex here. Press gently at first, as it can be tender. If you get no response, check that you are in the centre of the toe print and then press harder, then release.

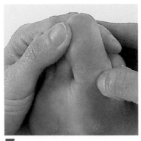

**7** Work around the neck of the big toe in two semi-circles: thumb-walk the back first.

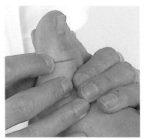

**8** Fingerwalk around the front of the big toe, using your index finger.

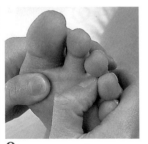

**9** For the smaller toes, follow the same routine as for the big toe. These toes can be covered in one line to each surface. Thumbwalk up the back.

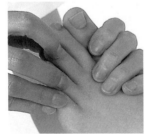

**10** Fingerwalk down the front of each toe to its base.

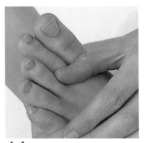

**11** Thumbwalk up one side of the toe. Always approach the side from the front. Change hands and work up the other side of the same toe.

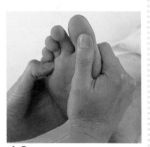

**12** Finally, thumbwalk the ridge under the little toes.

THE CHEST

The chest area is contained on the ball of the foot and on the top of the foot.

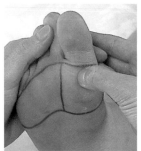
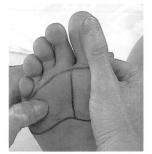
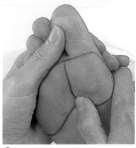
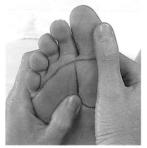

**1** Thumbwalk horizontally in from the instep under the big toe in zone 1 (for the five zones, see the illustrations on the head, neck and torso zones in the How Reflexology Works section), starting just next to the neck. Repeat just below the first line, bordering on it. Continue thumbwalking lines like this until you have covered the ball under the big toe down to the diaphragm line.

**2** Thumbwalk horizontally in from the outside of the foot under the little toes, starting just below the ridge. Cover the whole of this area in the same way as described in step 1.

**3** Next work along the diaphragm line under the big toe and follow the natural line up between the big and second toes to the base of the toes.

**4** Work along the diaphragm line from the outside, and when you meet the line between the big and second toes continue up this line to the base of the toes.

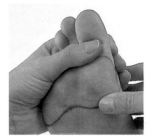
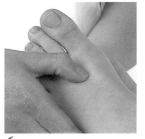
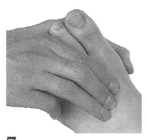

**5** Starting from just under the big toe, thumbwalk the whole diaphragm line.

**6** On the top of the foot, fingerwalk each channel between the bones leading to the toes.

**7** Use the three middle fingers together to fingerwalk the whole of the top of the foot, working from the base of the toes up the foot.

THE ABDOMEN

This area lies in the instep, starting under the diaphragm line and going down to the heel line.

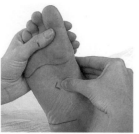 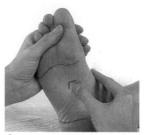 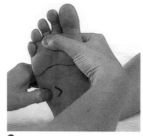 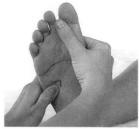

**1** Thumbwalk from the medial edge, under the big toe, out to the outer edge in horizontal lines as you did for the chest, each line bordering the previous one.

**2** Next thumbwalk diagonal lines covering the same area, as described in step 1.

**3** Now change hands and thumbwalk horizontal lines from the outside of the foot to the inner (medial) edge, as before.

**4** Finally, with the same thumb, thumbwalk diagonal lines from the outside to the inner edge covering the whole area, as before.

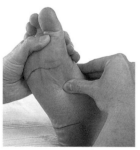 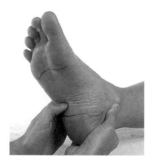 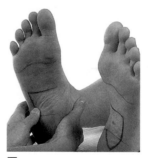 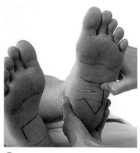

**5** Referring to the foot chart at the back of the book, gently rotate the reflex to the adrenal glands, pushing in under the tendon running down from the big toe.

**6** Work the ileo-caecal valve reflex, using the inner corner of your thumb to pinpoint it.

**7** Thumbwalk the path of the colon, starting on the right foot at the bottom of the colon line.

**8** Continue on to the left foot, following the line as outlined on the foot chart at the back of the book. Change from left hand to right hand at the point above.

THE PELVIS

The pelvic area lies all around the heel: on the sole, the sides of the heel and on top of the ankle.

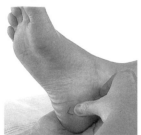

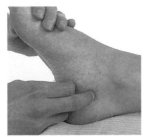

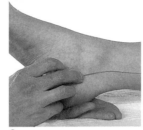

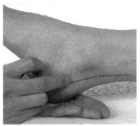

**1** Thumbwalk the heel across the sole in horizontal, overlapping lines. (This is hard work.)

**2** Find the little hollow halfway along a diagonal line between the centre of the ankle bone and the right angle of the heel on the inside of the foot, and rotate this point with your middle fingertip. Do not apply too much pressure.

**3** From this point, fingerwalk with the same finger up the line running behind the ankle up the leg.

**4** Now find the point described in step 2, but on the outside of the foot. Rotate it with the middle finger of your other hand and then fingerwalk up the outside of the ankle and leg, just as you did on the inside.

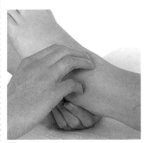

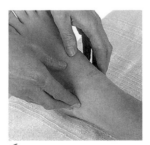

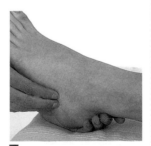

THE LIMBS

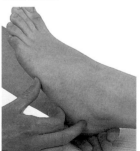

**5** Using the three middle fingers, fingerwalk across the top of the ankle.

**6** Continue round the ankle bone with the same fingertips.

**7** Refer to the foot charts to find the hip/knee reflex, and work it by fingerwalking two fingers together.

**1** Work the outside of the foot, then massage the relevant cross reflex.

# THE SEQUENCES

When you have learnt, and feel comfortable with, the whole routine for giving reflexology you may begin to pay special attention to certain reflexes for specific reasons, as you work. Always work the reflex on both feet unless the right or left foot is specified.

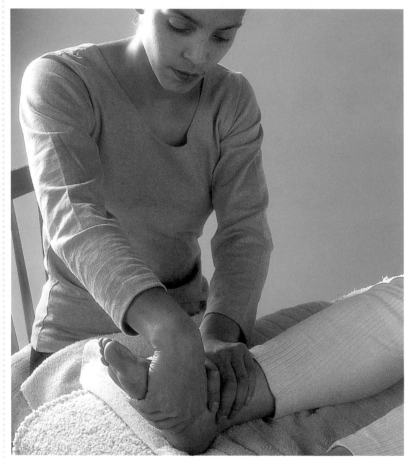

When giving reflexology you must always be sensitive to the response, particularly to painful or congested areas.

## HOW TO USE THE SEQUENCES WITHIN THE WHOLE ROUTINE

If you are giving reflexology at the end of the day, for instance, to relax someone and promote a good night's sleep, when you get to the reflex for the diaphragm you will be aware that it is particularly beneficial to work that part in order to assist relaxation and rest, and so you will work with special awareness and sensitivity there.

In giving special attention to certain reflexes you may feel drawn to do more massage in that place, or you may find the reflex is tender and you need to work more gently and perhaps for a little longer to release some of the tension felt there. Or you may stop to rotate on the reflex gently where you would otherwise simply have covered the area by thumbwalking.

Your way of working must be dictated by the response of your partner, taking into account how they feel, how they are experiencing the massage and what they and you can feel on their feet.

### WHAT TO DO IF YOUR PARTNER FEELS IT IS PAINFUL

Finding congestion or tenderness on the reflexes is never a reason for enthusiastic working at a specific reflex for an extended period, and you must never ever work if you are causing pain. In this situation massage gently, instead of thumbwalking, and then, if you are able to continue on the tender spot without causing discomfort, do so by working more gently to ensure that you do no harm. The golden rule is that you always take your lead from the person you are working with: follow what they are telling you about where they hurt and where they can take more or less of your touch.

Do not go to the other extreme and miss out parts that hurt, however, as they are just the places that need anything which will assist or stimulate them to heal themselves. Your job is to work out how best you may assist this process and if this means that all you can do without causing pain and discomfort is to hold the

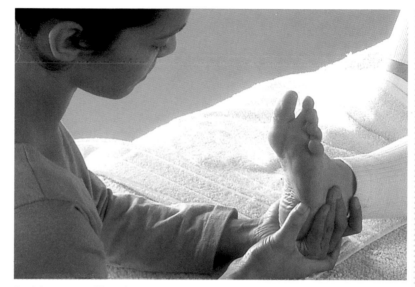

Position yourself so that you are comfortable and have a good view of the soles of the feet.

troubled part gently, or just stroke it with a fingertip, do so.

As long as you listen to your partner, to what they say and to their body language, and take your approach from what they and their feet are telling you, you will be doing well.

If you have not yet read the introduction to this section please read it now before going any further, to make sure that you do no harm. Your treatment of the feet will stimulate and balance all the body systems and you are now

ready to incorporate the sequences that follow, if you wish to highlight specific areas.

CAUTION
Working any of the following sequences in isolation, without working the whole foot routine, will not be effective and may cause damage. These sequences are for you to add to the basic routine as you work through it.

# RELAXATION SEQUENCES
## AIDING RESTFUL SLEEP

You will benefit more from a night's sleep if your body is relaxed and tense muscles loosened before you go to bed. Otherwise you may wake stiff, in pain, with a headache or unrefreshed; or you may wake during the night and be unable to get back to sleep.

Through massage and stimulating the reflexes you will improve the circulation and this, in turn, will accelerate the body's removal of waste. In this way you are doing what you can to enhance the systems of the body and to enable it to make the most of the healing properties of sleep.

It is important to use plenty of massage on your partner's feet during the routine. Always include ankle rotation, as this loosens tension there. All the blood supply and nerves to the feet pass through the ankles, and so it is very important that these flow freely, unrestricted by excessive tension.

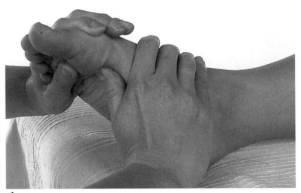

**1** To relax the diaphragm, hold the foot with your outside hand, bring it down on to the thumb of your other hand and lift it off again. Move your thumb one step to the side and repeat the movement, until you have worked your thumb across the foot to the outer side, following the boundary line of the ball of the foot where it meets the instep (the diaphragm line).

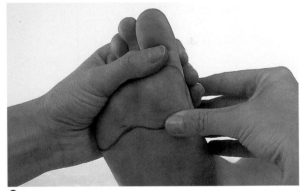

**2** Thumbwalk along the whole of the diaphragm line. Relaxing the diaphragm is especially important, as it helps to relax the whole body and to steady breathing.

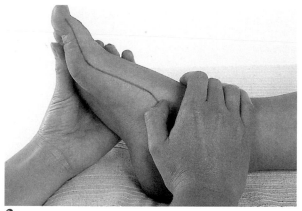

**3** Thumbwalk along the spinal reflex from the heel to the big toe. Always remember to support the foot. In this instance, support the outside of the foot with your other hand.

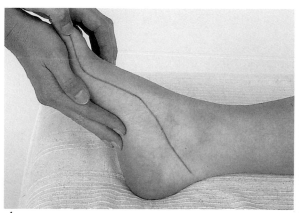

**4** Repeat the movement, going down the spinal reflex. Repeat up and down several times. Slow down to feel for any tight or sensitive parts and rotate gently around those spots.

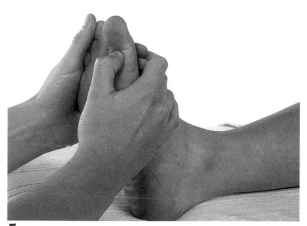

**5** Thumbwalk up the back of the toes: do this with care as there is likely to be a lot of tenderness there.

### SELF-HELP

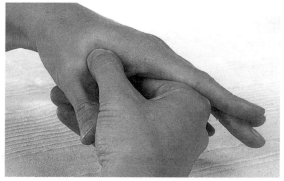

You can help to relax tension in yourself by massaging the web between your thumb and index finger on both hands.

# NECK AND SHOULDER RELAXERS

We collect much tension in our necks. If you are not aware of neck tension put your hands on either side of your neck and massage gently. If it feels tight or uncomfortable you may benefit from this sequence as your partner works your feet.

When neck muscles are tense and tight they constrict the nerves, which may in turn lead to pain, noises in the ears, or tired eyes. If you suffer from aching shoulders you will find that relaxing the tense shoulder muscles will not only relieve the aching but will improve your breathing as well. Tight shoulder muscles will pull your chest tight and consequently restrict your breathing.

Within the framework of the whole routine you may pay special attention to the following areas.

NECK TENSION

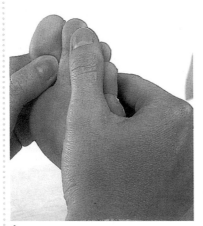

**1** Thumbwalk up the side of the neck on the big toe, where a lot of tension collects. Repeat this up the neck of all the toes and thumbwalk around the neck of the big toe, starting from the back.

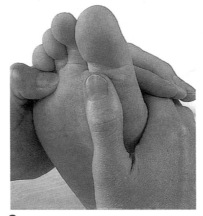

**2** Thumbwalk along the ridge immediately under the toes. Make sure you are right on top of this ridge, as it is easy to move below it, which will not have the same effect.

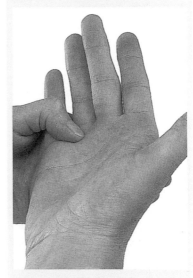

SELF–HELP

Thumbwalk along the base of your fingers.

SHOULDER TENSION

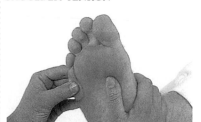

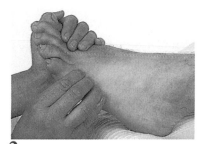

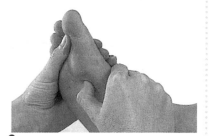

**1** If you are working with some-one who has shoulder tension, thumbwalk along the line of the shoulders in horizontal, overlapping lines.

**2** Fingerwalk across the same area on the top of the foot with three fingers. Then fingerwalk around the mid-back with three fingers, working in rows from the lower joint of the little toe down to the waistline (halfway down the foot).

**3** To relax the diaphragm, position your thumb on the diaphragm line underneath the big toe. Hold the foot with your out-side hand, bring it down on to the thumb of your other hand and lift it off again. Move your thumb one step to the outer side of the foot and repeat the movement, until you have worked your thumb across the foot to the outer side, following the boundary line of the ball of the foot where it meets the instep (the diaphragm line).

SELF-HELP
Thumbwalk and massage around the shoulder line on your hands (refer to the hand chart at the back of the book).

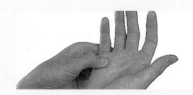

WHIPLASH INJURIES

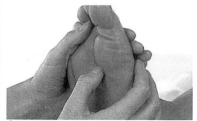

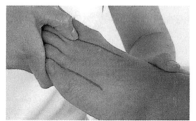

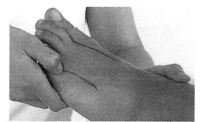

**1** Thumbwalk the first channel, between the big and second toes.

**2** Work the same area on the top of the feet with your thumb.

**3** Work the shoulder reflex on the top and the bottom of the feet.

# BACKACHE RELIEVERS

Backache is draining, both from the constant aching and because it saps your strength as it constricts your central nervous system (in the spinal cord). More working days are lost through backache than from any other cause. Release tension and relax the supporting muscles in the following areas.

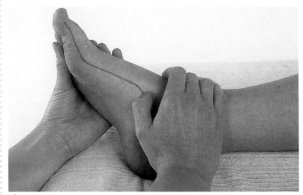

**1** Thumbwalk up and down the spine, supporting the outer edge of the foot as you work.

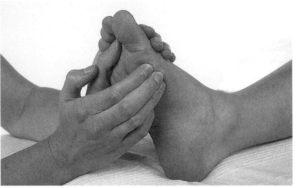

**2** Fingerwalk across the spinal reflex with three fingers together, right down the instep in stripes.

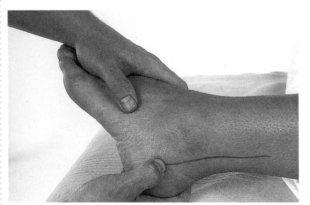

**3** Thumbwalk up the helper reflexes for the lower back, behind the ankle bones on either side.

SELF-HELP

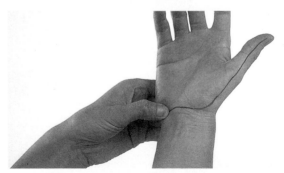

Work the spinal reflex on your hands.

# RELIEVING REPETITIVE STRAIN

If you work at a computer for long periods you may suffer from eye strain, or your wrists may ache and hurt from using the keyboard. Any desk job may give you stiff shoulders and a stiff neck. If you are on your feet all day you may well end the day with tired and swollen legs and ankles, and sore feet. The best way to relieve all this strain is to work the whole feet so that the various systems will be stimulated to function more efficiently. In addition you can choose whichever of the following are appropriate.

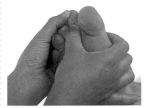

**1** Thumbwalk up the back and sides of the second and third toes for the eye reflex. This will also relieve neck tension.

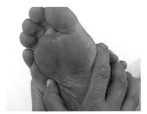

**2** Work the shoulder reflexes thoroughly by using the thumbwalking technique.

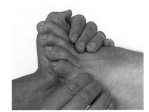

**3** Fingerwalk across the same area on the top of the foot, with the three middle fingers together.

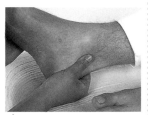

**4** Rotate the ankles to ease aching wrists and stimulate healing within the joints.

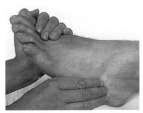

**5** Work across and down the outer foot on both feet to relax shoulders, arms, legs and knees.

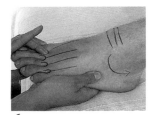

**6** Work the lymph system on both feet. Fingerwalk down the lines from the toes towards the ankle. Then work around the ankle.

### SELF-HELP

Use the hand chart at the back of the book to find the relevant reflex on your hands to give temporary, quick relief for your particular problem. The point to remember when dealing with repetitive strain is that there is no one sequence of movements to help. It is up to you to work out which part of your body is suffering from the strain and locate the relevant reflex from the hand and foot charts that are located at the back of the book.

# ENLIVENING MUSCLES

Rather than going from one extreme to another and trying to compensate for a sedentary job by doing vigorous exercise with a sluggish body, get someone to give you a foot treatment stimulating the circulation and all the bodily systems. You may then really feel like doing something energetic the next day, because you will feel so much better. You will also benefit more from exercise if your body is not being forced. If you are doing this for someone else, concentrate on the following areas in your full treatment.

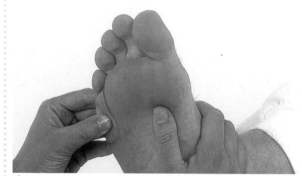

**1** Thumbwalk along the line of the shoulders.

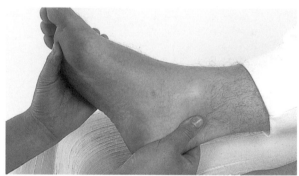

**2** Rotate the ankles to loosen tension and increase the circulation and to ease pressure on the nerve supply.

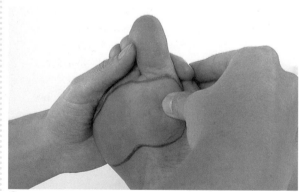

**3** Work the whole of the chest and lung area.

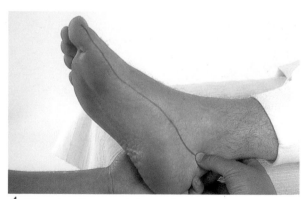

**4** Thumbwalk up and down the spine.

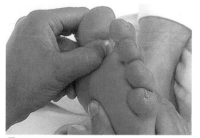

**5** Starting with the big toe, work the neck on all the toes.

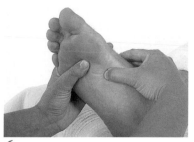

**6** Rotate the adrenal reflex gently. This will stimulate it to respond as your body's natural sense directs: to relax and aid recovery from overwork or to stimulate in readiness for activity.

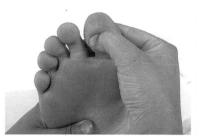

**7** Rotate or massage gently on all the reflexes to other important endocrine glands, which regulate the chemicals in your body and therefore your bodily activity.

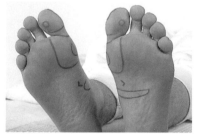

**8** Pinpoint the pituitary reflex in the big toe. Thumbwalk the thyroid helper on the ball of the foot. Rotate the adrenals and work the pancreas on the instep.

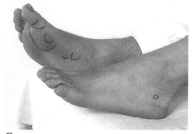

**9** Rotate on the ovaries/testes reflex at the side of the heel.

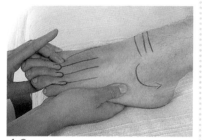

**10** Thumbwalk or rotate (as appropriate) the reflexes of the lymph system.

# STRESS RELIEVERS

Excessive stress lies somewhere behind most troubles and illness. If your adrenalin runs at a high level for long periods, with little chance of appropriate action, your adrenal glands will become depleted. Your breathing will either become too rapid or will be restricted and shallow. Your digestion will be upset or strained in some way. If you feel nervous or queasy the first thing to do is to breathe more deeply and slowly. This will calm you down, settle your nerves and increase the supply of oxygen to your body. It is not possible to panic while you are breathing well. Help the calming process by working on your hands, massaging with your thumb the solar plexus reflex in your palms. Do this on both hands. If you are giving a reflexology treatment pay special attention to the following areas.

### RELIEVING GENERAL STRESS

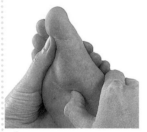 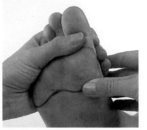 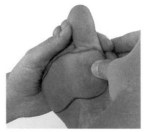 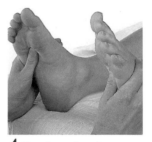

**1** Relax the diaphragm: hold the foot with your outside hand, bring it down on to the thumb of your other hand and lift it off again. Move your thumb one step to the outer side and repeat the movement, until you have worked your thumb across the foot, following the boundary line of the ball of the foot.

**2** Thumbwalk along the diaphragm line. Tension collects in the diaphragm, causing pain and tightness. When the diaphragm is contracting and relaxing freely the abdominal organs are stimulated also.

**3** Work the lung reflexes on the chest area so that once the diaphragm is relaxed, breathing can be increased. This will help you to relax, get the oxygen you need and promote well-being.

**4** Do the solar plexus breathing exercise: take both feet together and position your thumbs in the centre of the diaphragm line. As your partner breathes in, press in with your thumbs, and release as they breathe out. Repeat several times following your partner's lead so that it is a comfortable rhythm for them.

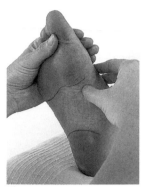

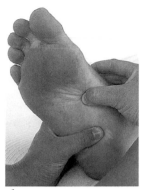

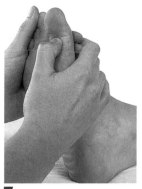

SELF-HELP

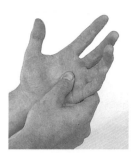

**5** Thumbwalk the stomach area and the whole of the instep, which is the abdominal area. This will help digestion and elimination, which are both affected by stress.

**6** Rotate gently on the adrenal reflex.

**7** Work the neck reflex on the neck of the toes where stress and tension collect.

Massage the centre of your palms, including the solar plexus reflex.

NERVOUS STOMACH OR "BUTTERFLIES"
Work the self-help areas illustrated above right, or steps 4 and 5 for someone to whom you are giving a full treatment.

STRESS FROM ANGER

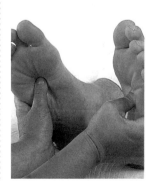

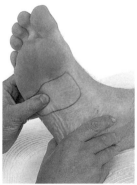

SELF-HELP
Referring to the hand charts at the back of the book, work the solar plexus reflexes and the liver area on your hands for self-help.

**1** Work the solar plexus reflexes on both feet.

**2** Work the liver area.

# ENHANCING SEQUENCES

If you have not yet read the introduction to the sequences please read it now, before you begin, to make sure that you do no harm. Within a treatment covering the whole of the feet, and so stimulating all the bodily systems, you may choose to pay special attention to the following specific areas.

## STARTING THE DAY: STIMULATING THE SYSTEMS AND THE SENSES

To make the most of your potential, your bodily systems need to be functioning well as you start the day and to continue to do so throughout the day.

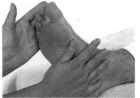 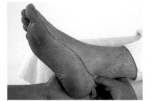 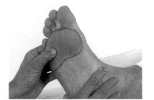 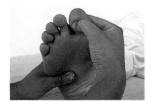

**1** Give some good vigorous massage to the whole feet to get the circulation going. Massage the chest area especially to help establish good breathing. Massage the instep using effleurage to stimulate the nervous system in the spinal cord and "wake up" the spine and its supporting muscles.

**2** Thumbwalk the spine. Rotate the ankles and the toes to stimulate the circulation to the feet and loosen the neck and pelvis, thus freeing the nerves to the head and lower body.

**3** Work the diaphragm, and then work across the chest. This will help to establish deep and regular, steady breathing to strengthen your body.

**4** Work the pituitary reflex on the big toe in the centre of the toe-print: this is the master gland and its functioning controls the other endocrine glands and your bodily systems in many ways.

SELF-HELP

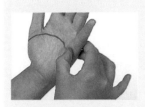

**1** To get yourself going at the beginning of the day, work the diaphragm on your hands.

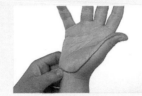

**2** Work the spine. Finally, work the pituitary reflex, which is located in the centre of your thumb-print.

# IMPROVING DECISIVENESS

When your body is tired and functioning below par, getting through normal daily tasks and making decisions will often seem more difficult. The liver and gall bladder work together so that the body may be strong and planning and decision-making happen naturally. By working the diaphragm, solar plexus and liver you are enhancing good breathing which strengthens the body.

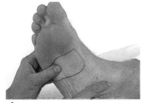

**1** Work the liver.

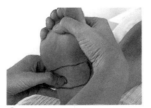

**2** Work the gall bladder.

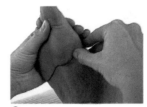

**3** Work the diaphragm.

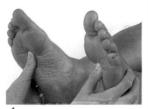

**4** Work the solar plexus.

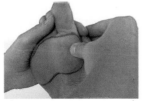

**5** Work the lungs.

SELF-HELP
Locate the gall bladder reflex on your right hand and rotate on it to aid decisiveness.

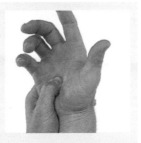

# ENERGY LEVEL ENHANCERS

If energy is flowing freely around your body you will feel well and find it easier to feel positive. In turn, if you think positively your body will respond and its actions will be enhanced. The power of thought influences your physical well-being and, conversely, your moods are much affected by your hormonal balance and the general well-being of your body.

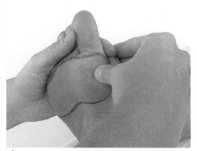

**1** Work the lungs to improve your breathing.

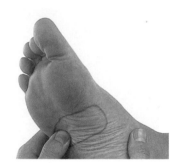

**2** Work the liver, the many functions of which are crucial to your general health.

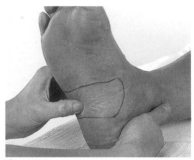

**3** Work the small intestines to aid the uptake of nutrients.

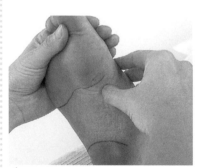

**4** Work the whole digestive area. What you eat is turned into your energy during digestion.

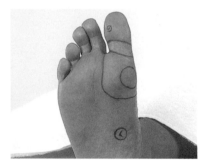

**5** Work the glands. Find the pituitary gland on the big toe. Work the thyroid on the neck of the big toe and the ball under it. Rotate the adrenals.

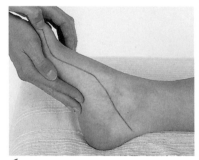

**6** Work up and down the spine, which is your central column of energy flow.

## SELF-HELP

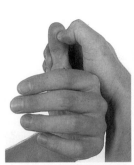 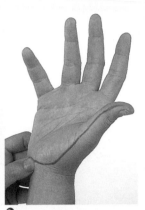 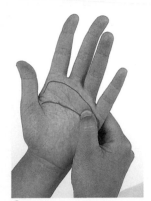 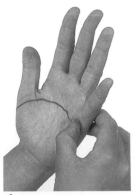

**1** Work the pituitary reflex in the centre of the thumb-print.

**2** Work the spinal reflex on the hands.

**3** Work the lungs to enhance breathing.

**4** Work the diaphragm on the hands.

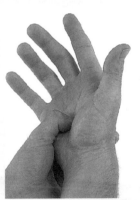 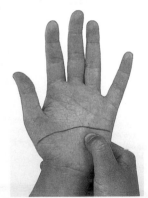 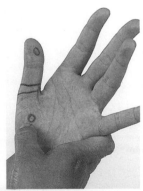

**5** Work the liver reflex on your right hand.

**6** Work the small intestines.

**7** Work the main glands to balance the hormonal system.

# IMPROVING SKIN, HAIR AND NAIL CONDITION

To keep your skin, hair and nails in good condition you need hormone balance, good nutrition and effective removal of toxins through the excretory system. Stimulation of the circulation through giving a whole reflexology treatment will aid the removal of toxins from the body and the supply of nutrients through the bloodstream; but remember that the supply of nutrients to your body will only be as good as those you put in through the food you eat. Good health is only possible if you eat a well-balanced mixture of good, "live" food. Poor health will result from processed food which is precooked and then reheated as it has little quality in it.

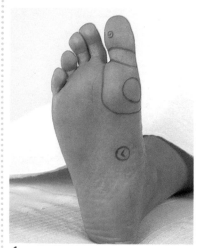

**1** Work all the glands on both feet. Your skin, hair and nails are kept in good health by chemicals in your hormones, which are controlled by your glands.

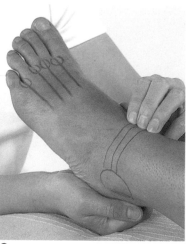

**2** In addition, make sure that you give attention to the lymph system on both feet to help remove toxins from the body.

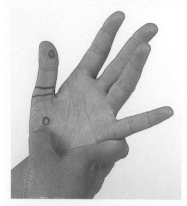

SELF-HELP

Work all the glands on your hands by referring to the hand chart at the back of the book.

# STRENGTHENING THE IMMUNE SYSTEM

Where the immune system is strong, the body will deal naturally with threatening infections so that they cannot become established. Within the context of a full reflexology routine, pay particular attention to the following areas.

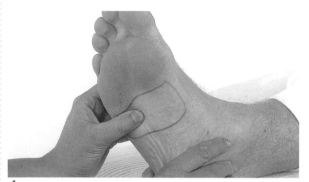

**1** Work the liver to strengthen the whole body.

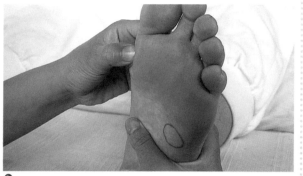

**2** Work the spleen (marked on the left foot) and rotate the thymus gland (on both feet) where the thumb is positioned in the above photograph.

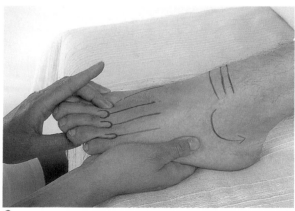

**3** Work the upper and lower lymph systems on both feet to aid the removal of toxins.

### SELF-HELP

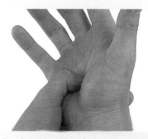

Work the liver and spleen to strengthen your body, and the thymus and lymph to fight off imminent infection. See the hand chart at the back of the book.

# RELIEVING SEQUENCES

If you have not yet read the introduction to the sequences please read it now, before you go any further, to make sure that you do no harm. Within a treatment covering the whole of the feet, and so stimulating all the bodily systems, you may choose to pay special attention to the following areas.

## PAIN RELIEVERS

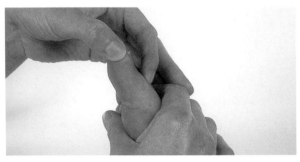

Before concentrating on the specific area of pain, work the hypothalamus reflex: the hypothalamus controls the release of endorphins for the relief of pain.

PAINFUL MUSCLES OR JOINTS

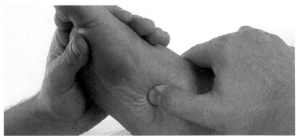

**1** Work the adrenal gland reflexes on both feet. These glands deal with inflammation and aid good muscle tone when working effectively.

BACK PAIN

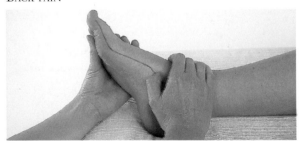

**1** Work along the spine and find the tender parts. Work these to try to disperse some of the congestion.

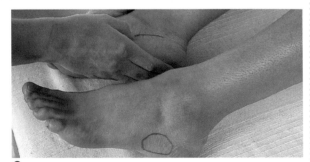

**2** For lower back trouble, work the helper area for this by rotating with your thumb.

NERVE PAIN

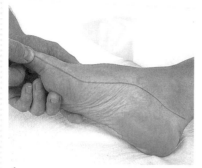

**1** Thumbwalk along the spine for the central nervous system in the spinal cord.

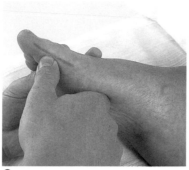

**2** Find the local area: for example, for the neck, work the cervical vertebrae and find the part of the neck of the toes that is tender.

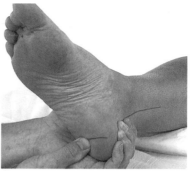

**3** For sciatic pain, work the sciatic reflex as shown in the foot chart at the back of the book.

CRAMP

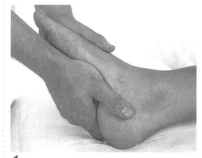

**1** Hold the area and massage the appropriate cross reflex. For example, for cramp in the calf, massage the cross reflex on the lower arm.

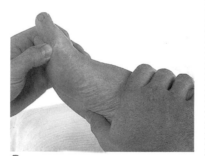

**2** Work the parathyroid reflexes round the neck of the big toe.

TOOTHACHE

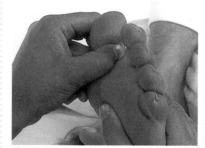

**1** Find the toe or finger that has much tenderness and work that area carefully but thoroughly.

# SLEEP ENHANCERS

There are many different reasons for insomnia and different manifestations of it. Do you have difficulty in getting to sleep or do you wake during the night and find you cannot get back to sleep? Do you feel the trouble is digestive or are you a worrier? (These two problems may be linked.)
You can help to promote a good night's sleep with this sequence.

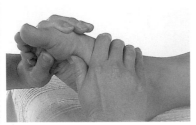

**1** To relax the diaphragm hold the foot with your outside hand, bring it down on to the thumb of your other hand and lift it off again. Move your thumb one step to the side and repeat the movement, until you have worked your thumb all the way across the foot to the outer side, following the diaphragm line.

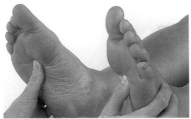

**2** Do the solar plexus breathing exercise: take both feet together and position your thumbs in the centre of the diaphragm line. As your partner breathes in, press gently in with your thumbs, and, as they breathe out, release. Repeat this several times following your partner's lead so that it is a comfortable rhythm for them.

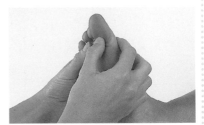

**3** Work the neck on all the toes to remove any tension that has built up in the neck muscles.

### SELF-HELP

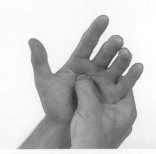

For self-help gently massage the solar plexus reflex in the palms of your hands.

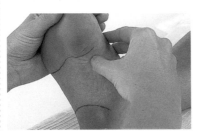

**4** Work the abdominal reflexes to relieve tension there.

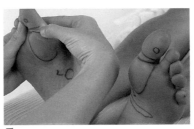

**5** Work all the glands, for good hormonal balance.

# BREATHING RELIEVERS

Respiratory problems may include hayfever and allergic reactions. Poor diet, pollution, excessive toxins in the body and excessive stress all undermine the body's strength and may cause a problem in the respiratory system.

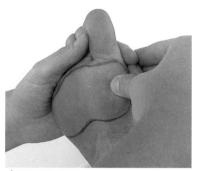

**1** Work the whole chest area on bottom of the feet to relieve the chest and lungs.

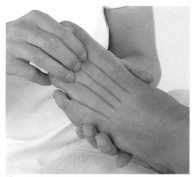

**2** Fingerwalk the same area on the top of the feet to stimulate the chest lymph.

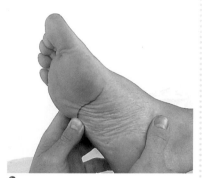

**3** Work the diaphragm to promote good breathing.

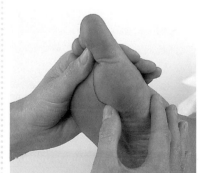

**4** Work the air passages to stimulate them to clear themselves.

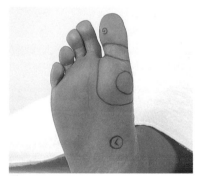

**5** Work all the glands and take particular notice of any that seem especially tender.

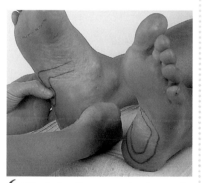

**6** Work the ileo-caecal valve and the whole of the colon because this will help balance mucus levels and get rid of waste in the system.

# RELIEVING HEADACHES AND NAUSEA

These two problems are often linked, with a blinding headache often contributing to feelings of nausea. Within the context of a full reflexology treatment, work for one or both as appropriate.

HEADACHES

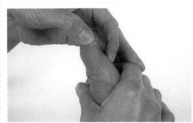

**1** Work the hypothalamus reflex first, as this controls the release of endorphins for the relief of pain.

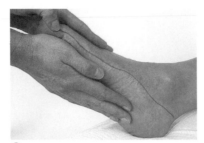

**2** Work down the spine to take pressure away from the head. This will draw energy down the body and ground it.

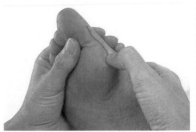

**3** Work the cervical spine on the big toe. Work the neck of all the toes to relieve tension.

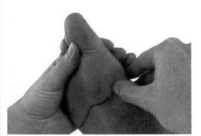

**4** Work the diaphragm to encourage breathing.

NAUSEA

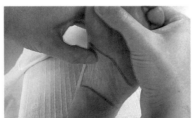

**1** Work the whole abdomen, especially where it seems tender. Do this gently and with care.

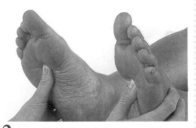

**2** Do the solar plexus breathing exercise: take both feet together and position your thumbs in the centre of the diaphragm line. As your partner breathes in, press gently in with your thumbs, and, as they breathe out, release your thumbs. Repeat this several times following your partner's lead.

# HELP WITH MENSTRUAL AND REPRODUCTIVE PROBLEMS

Work the whole reproductive system on the sides and top of the heel, as all parts work together.

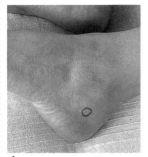 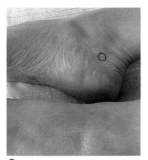 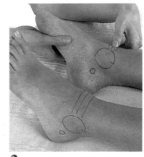

**1** Work the ovaries or testes on the outside of the feet.

**2** Work the uterus or prostate gland on the inside of the feet.

**3** Work the fallopian tubes or vas deferens across the top of the ankle.

SELF-HELP
Refer to the hand chart at the back of the book to locate the ovaries or testes, and work this reflex on both hands. Then work the uterus or prostate gland, and finally the fallopian tubes or vas deferens.

MENSTRUAL CRAMPS

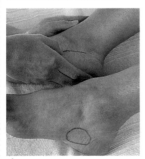 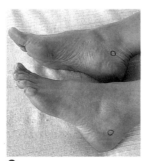 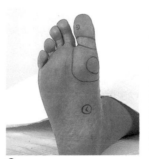

PAINFUL BREASTS

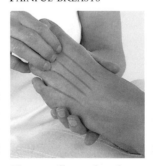

**1** Work the lower spine for nerves to the uterus.

**2** Work the uterus reflex on the inside of the feet.

**3** Work the glands on both feet.

Fingerwalk up the chest area on top of the foot with three fingers together.

# HELP WITH COLDS, SORE THROATS AND SINUS PROBLEMS

Colds, sore throats and sinus problems all affect the respiratory system. To stimulate them to clear themselves, you need to work all the toes and chest area.

COLDS

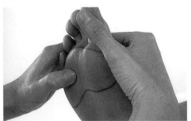

**1** Work the chest to encourage clear breathing.

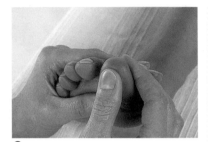

**2** Beginning with the big toe, work the tops of all the toes to clear the sinuses. Then pinpoint the pituitary gland in the centre of the prints of both big toes to stimulate the endocrine system.

SORE THROATS

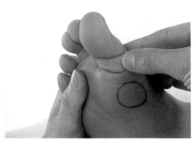

**1** Work the upper lymph system, and then work the throat on the neck, and the thymus gland for the immune system.

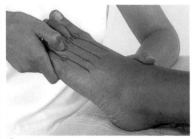

**3** Work the upper lymph system to stimulate the immune system.

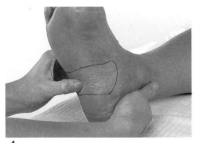

**4** Work the small intestines to aid elimination of toxins and uptake of nutrients. Then work the colon to aid elimination.

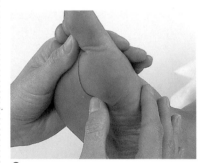

**2** Work the trachea and the larynx to stimulate them to clear and heal.

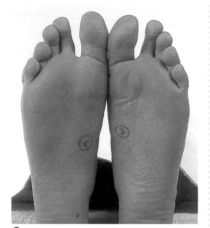

**3** Rotate the adrenal reflex in the direction of the arrow.

SINUS PROBLEMS

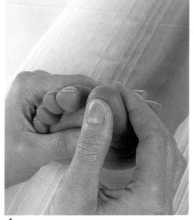

**1** Work all the toes, especially the sinus reflexes to stimulate them to clear themselves.

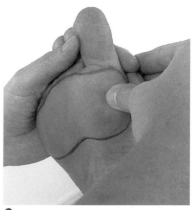

**2** Work the whole chest area to aid respiration.

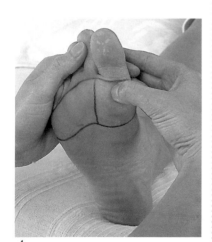

**4** Work the thyroid helper area in the section of the chest under the big toe. Then work the whole chest area for the entire respiratory system.

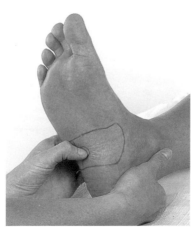

**3** Pinpoint the ileo-caecal valve to balance mucus levels.

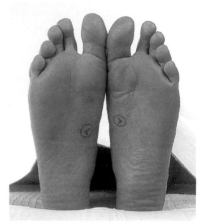

**4** Rotate the adrenal reflex to reduce inflammation.

# IMPROVING THE DIGESTION

The digestive system is a complex one with many and varied functions. It can be easily affected by stress and tension and, in the context of a full reflexology routine, particular attention can be given to the following areas.

INDIGESTION

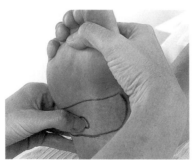

**1** Work the solar plexus to relax the nerves to the stomach.

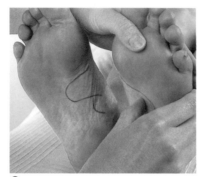

**2** Work the stomach, where digestion really begins.

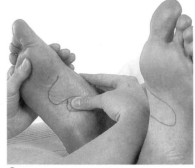

**3** Then work the duodenum, the first section of the small intestines.

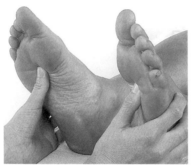

**4** Work the liver and the gall bladder: the liver area is shown above, with the thumb rotating on the gall bladder reflex. These deal with digestion of fats.

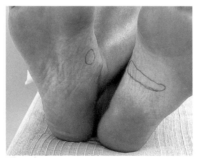

**5** Work the pancreas which regulates blood sugar levels and aids digestion.

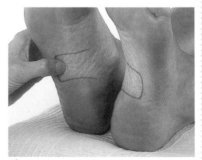

**6** Work the small intestines where nutrients are absorbed. If there is bloatedness work the colon. (See the sequence for constipation opposite.)

CONSTIPATION

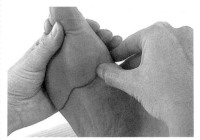

**1** Work the diaphragm to relax the abdomen.

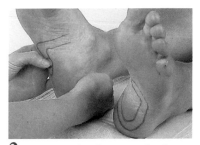

**2** Pinpoint the ileo-caecal valve, which links small and large intestines.

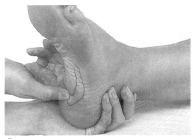

**3** Work the colon or large intestine, especially the descending and sigmoid colon. This can become congested.

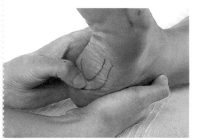

**4** Pinpoint the sigmoid flexure. Being a bend, this can become congested.

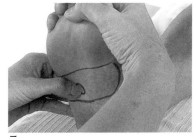

**5** Work the liver and gall bladder: the liver area is shown above, with the thumb rotating on the gall bladder reflex.

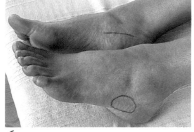

**6** Work the lower spine and its helper areas for the nerve supply to the colon.

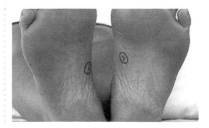

**7** Work the adrenals for muscle tone. Rotate the reflex with your thumb in the direction of the arrows.

SELF-HELP
Work the diaphragm to relax the abdomen and work the reflexes as described for the feet.

# FOOT CHARTS

The foot charts are only guidelines for interpretation. When you find a tender or congested part of the foot you may look for that part on the charts and see approximately which reflex the tenderness lies on. This is only a rough guide because every pair of feet are different and will not be the same shape as your chart. Also, the charts are two-dimensional and your body is three-dimensional and therefore the reflexes on your feet reflect this. In reality your organs overlap each other, whereas the charts are much simplified for clarity, to give an idea of where things are.

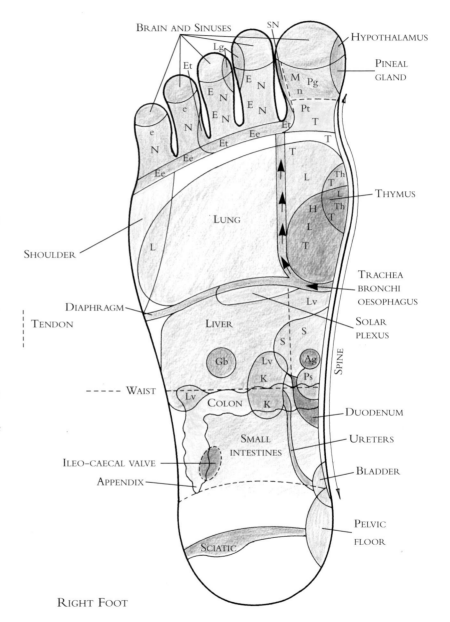

BRAIN AND SINUSES
SN
HYPOTHALAMUS
PINEAL GLAND
THYMUS
TRACHEA BRONCHI OESOPHAGUS
SOLAR PLEXUS
SPINE
DUODENUM
URETERS
BLADDER
PELVIC FLOOR

SHOULDER
DIAPHRAGM
TENDON
WAIST
ILEO-CAECAL VALVE
APPENDIX

Lung
LIVER
COLON
SMALL INTESTINES
SCIATIC

RIGHT FOOT

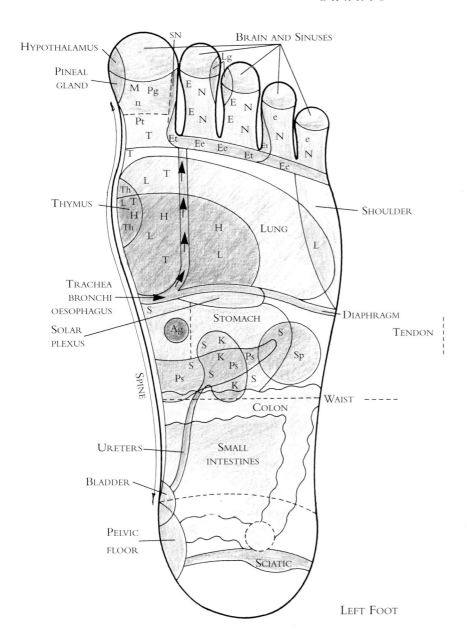

HYPOTHALAMUS

PINEAL
GLAND

SN

BRAIN AND SINUSES

Lg

M Pg
n

Pt

T

T

THYMUS

Th
L T
L T
T H
L Th
L

T

E
N
E
N
Et

E
N
E
N
Ee

E
N
E
N
Ee

e
N
Et

e
N
Ee

Et

SHOULDER

TRACHEA
BRONCHI
OESOPHAGUS

SOLAR
PLEXUS

SPINE

T
L

H

L

T

L

LUNG

L

S

Ag

STOMACH

S K
K
S Ps
Ps
S
Ps S K

S

Sp

S

DIAPHRAGM

TENDON

WAIST

COLON

URETERS

BLADDER

PELVIC
FLOOR

SMALL
INTESTINES

SCIATIC

LEFT FOOT

KEY

Ag Adrenal glands

e Ears

Et Eustachian tubes

Ee Eye/Ear helper

E Eyes

Gb Gall bladder

H Heart

K Kidneys

Lg Lachrymal glands

Lv Liver

L Lungs

M Mouth

N Neck

n Nose

Ps Pancreas

Pt Para-thyroid

Pg Pituitary glands

SN Side of neck

Sp Spleen

S Stomach

Tb Trachea bronchi oesophagus

th Thymus

T Thyroid

# TOP AND SIDES OF FOOT

The spinal reflex (bottom) is especially important and should always be massaged, and the reflex worked thoroughly. Not only is our spinal column our main boney support but it also contains the spinal cord, and through the central nervous system the whole body may be treated on the spinal reflex.

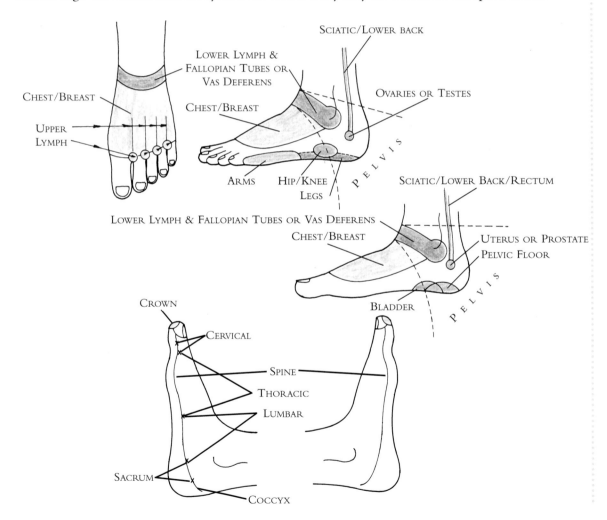

# HAND CHART

The hands reflect all the body, as do the feet. They are a very different shape to feet, but once you have adjusted to that and learnt the basic layout, the location of reflexes is quite straightforward. Use the reflexes on the hand when you cannot work the feet for any reason. This may be the accessibility of hands rather than feet, or damage or disease to the feet, for example.

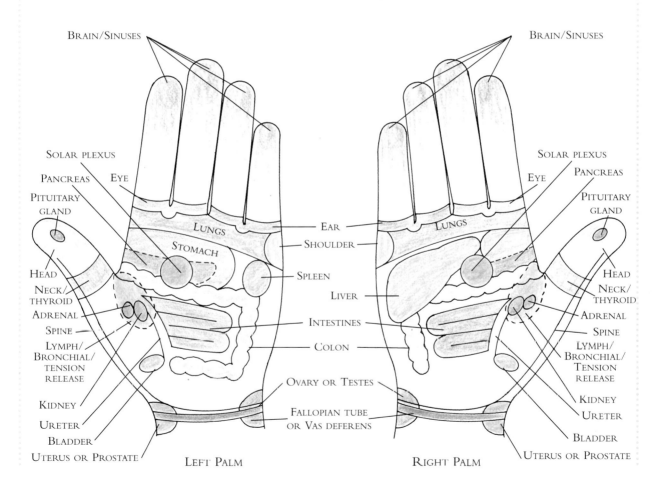

BRAIN/SINUSES

SOLAR PLEXUS
PANCREAS
EYE
PITUITARY GLAND
LUNGS
STOMACH
HEAD
NECK/ THYROID
ADRENAL
SPINE
LYMPH/ BRONCHIAL/ TENSION RELEASE
KIDNEY
URETER
BLADDER
UTERUS OR PROSTATE
LEFT PALM

BRAIN/SINUSES

SOLAR PLEXUS
PANCREAS
EYE
PITUITARY GLAND
LUNGS
EAR
SHOULDER
SPLEEN
LIVER
INTESTINES
COLON
OVARY OR TESTES
FALLOPIAN TUBE OR VAS DEFERENS
HEAD
NECK/ THYROID
ADRENAL
SPINE
LYMPH/ BRONCHIAL/ TENSION RELEASE
KIDNEY
URETER
BLADDER
UTERUS OR PROSTATE
RIGHT PALM

63

# INDEX

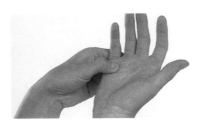

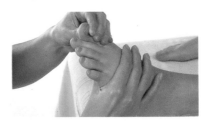